Fitness for Beginners Health & Wellness:

Exercise Benefits

By Cathy Wilson
Copyright © 2013

Income Disclaimer

This book contains business strategies, marketing methods and other business advice that, regardless of my own results and experience, may not produce the same results (or any results) for you. I make absolutely no guarantee, expressed or implied, that by following the advice below you will make any money or improve current profits, as there are several factors and variables that come into play regarding any given business.

Primarily, results will depend on the nature of the product or business model, the conditions of the marketplace, the experience of the individual, and situations and elements that are beyond your control.

As with any business endeavor, you assume all risk related to investment and money based on your own discretion and at your own potential expense.

Liability Disclaimer

By reading this book, you assume all risks associated with using the advice given below, with a full understanding that you, solely, are responsible for anything that may occur as a result of putting this information into action in any way, and regardless of your interpretation of the advice.

You further agree that our company cannot be held responsible in any way for the success or failure of your business as a result of the information presented in this book. It is your responsibility to conduct your own due diligence regarding the safe and successful operation of your business if you intend to apply any of our information in any way to your business operations.

Terms of Use

You are given a non-transferable, "personal use" license to this book. You cannot distribute it or share it with other individuals.

Also, there are no resale rights or private label rights granted when purchasing this book. In other words, it's for your own personal use only.

Table of Contents

Fitness for Beginners Health & Wellness:

Exercise Benefits

By Cathy Wilson

Introduction

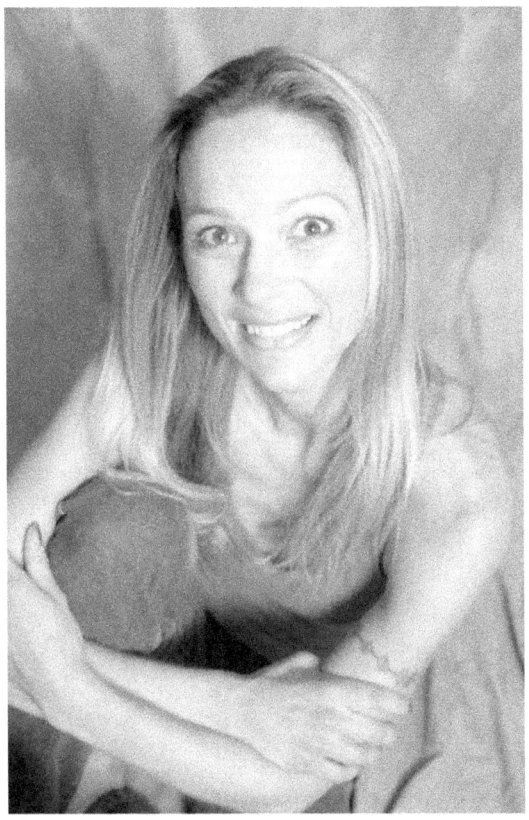

I have been fascinated with all aspects of nutrition, fitness, and overall health and wellness, since I started training for my first figure skating competition at the age of 7.

Since then, I've competed at a provincial level in 6 different sports and at "rep" level in 4 or 5 others. Through sweat, screwing up and determination, I've learned how to build a body and mind strong, safely. With all the mental, physical, and emotional components required to succeed. Whether you are looking to get off your dusty couch for the first time in years, or training for your second biathlon, Fitness for Beginners will help you.

My schooling is in nutrition, which has triggered my desire to learn more.

It's scary to think of the wealth of information and experiences I've accumulated over 30 years! Yikes - that dates me too, which is even scarier!

Semi-recently I've taken various training courses and loved the challenge of coaching people to better health, by creating unique exercise and nutritional programs built to get results fast that last.

The key is to make your new healthy choices habit, so they become your new "normal." Rather than a moment in time that gets tossed aside for comfort and familiarity. You've been there and done that, right? Just think fad diets and crazy exercise programs.

Currently I'm tuned into lean muscle building strategies, and fitness body building is on my list of things to do.

My want is to pass this wealth of knowledge that I have absorbed over 30 years onto you, or at least the parts you like to use.

Is there a specific reason for these books?

Yes. I can't count the number of great people that have asked my why I haven't published my own books on fitness, nutrition, health and wellness. These people, along with my 6 little ones have inspired me to write what I know.

Ask and you shall receive!

The reason I'm writing a series is because there are SO many factors involved in Fitness for Beginners alone, that it really does need to be broken down. This way you will gain a better base knowledge from which to build, without getting overwhelmed. Simple and effective is how it's gotta be.

The books are going to be . . .

* Book 1 - Exercise Benefits

* Book 2 - Pointers for Success in Nutrition and Fitness

* Book 3 - Getting Lean and Trim

* Book 4 - Eating For Energy

* Book 5 - Key to Weight Loss - Build Lean Muscle

. . . in Great Health, Fitness, and Positive Thinking.

Each of these factors is equally important in Fitness for Beginners.

I will give you the knowledge and practicality to set yourself up for success, and support you in this. One manageable step at a time and we WILL get you to the finish line with a smile and in better shape than you were yesterday.

Let's dig right into Book 1. Where we are going to learn all about the benefits of exercising and all that it "was" and is, why we exercise, how to get started, the different types of exercises, how you execute, and equipment that may help you. Your health matters and learning how to get fit and stay that way is only going to set you up to live a long, healthy, and happy life.

Exercise Benefits

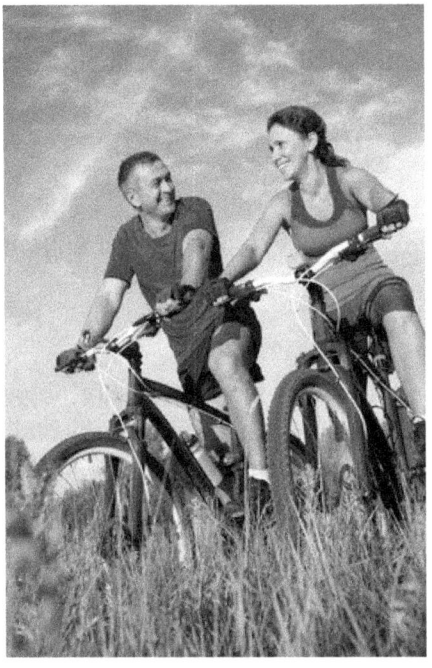

You are exercising when you go for a run, play an intense bump and grind basketball game, or just hike it up the stairs fast. It's that feeling of having to breathe deeper and longer. Sometimes even needing to stop a minute or two to catch your breath. That's your cardiovascular and muscles in action. Work it hard and regularly and you're going to increase your cardiovascular capacity and build lean muscle strength for better overall fitness. Never challenge your body, and with time you are going to notice the aches and pains more than if you were in better shape. Your energy levels will continually decline along with your positive perspective.

What is Cardiovascular specifically? We are going to start from the ground and work our way up,without getting too technically boring on you. Cardiovascular relates to the blood vessels and heart functioning, inclusive of veins and arteries. It's where you are participating in an exercise like running, that increases your heart rate and forces higher oxygen intake. Dynamic yoga, cycling, skating, rollerblading, circuits, swimming, and fast walking are great examples of cardiovascular exercise.

When aerobic activity is applied to exercise it's referred to as cardiovascular exercise. Which is often used as one factor in weight loss or conditioning training for athletes.

What is Muscle building? When you utilize your muscles during exercise, this builds muscle. In short, by weight training muscles you will build up your muscle cells and this is going to help your body burn more calories overall, by increasing your metabolism because muscle burns more calories than fat does. Muscle cells are also physically smaller than fat cells. So you have a smaller look. They are also firmer, so you aren't as "jiggly" as you would be with just fat cells.

FIT ALERT! Contrary to our programming of days past. Women don't need to be afraid they are going to end up looking like a muscle "hulkster" by weight training. Experts agree this is simply not true. A woman's body wasn't made with muscles cells that "normally" get as big as a man's.

Women don't have the hormonal makeup or the physical ability to get huge. Now if you are fooling around with hormones, specifically growth hormones, under the guidance of a trainer and doctor, you can force your body to build more muscle than the average woman would. But these women have a specific focus and are the exception to the rules. The best thing you can do for your body ladies is to start pumping iron!

Add muscle building or strength training to your cardiovascular exercise and you are going to build your body strong and efficient. Great at burning off excess calories and leaving you feel-feeling on top of the world!

My thinking . . . You can't have one without the other. If you want the maximum benefits from exercising you are going to need to get some your heart pumping and muscles working hard with regular aerobic exercise and muscle building strategies. Starting off with at least 30 minutes of cardio 3-4 days a week, and 2-3 days of muscle building for 15-20 minutes each time should do the trick. A solid platform from which to build.

I'm sure you've heard that everyone needs 30- 60 minutes of exercise each day to be healthy?

It's true and let me tell you why.

History of Exercise

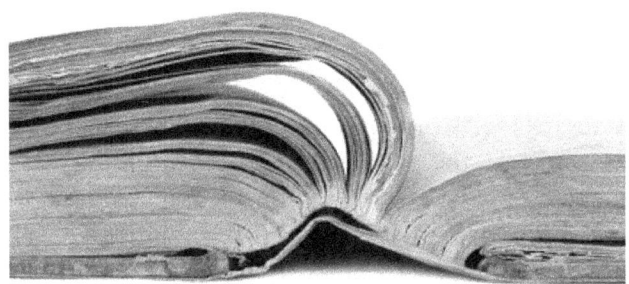

Exercise has been around since the beginning of time. Way back in ancient days, people had to be in fantastic cardiovascular shape or they didn't survive. Fittest of the fittest was a reality for them.

They lived differently and every single thing people did require physical exercise. Not like us today, where we don't even have to get out of bed to eat if we don't want to. Well that isn't quite true because you might have to get up to answer the door and pay the pizza delivery boy. Geesh!

People in the olden days had a full day of diverse exercise every time they wanted to eat. If they were lucky, they had a horse to hop on. They'd grab their bow and arrow or spear, and head off two miles into the bush to hunt for game. And if their tracking skills were bang on, they would find some tasty antelope or maybe a gazelle to bring down. So they would chase the game down, kill it, and then drag it two miles back to camp.

They weren't done yet! I think the women got the skinning and cleaning job. But the men would still have to head out to get firewood and anything else that may be required for the feast. If they were lucky a nap might work while the women were cooking up the all-natural protein based dinner. Sometime late in the day they would be ready to feast until all bellies were full. Only to wake up hungry the next morning, and out the men would go for another hunt.

You see these people didn't need to think of ways to make time to exercise themselves physically, mentally, and emotionally. They got all this in the hunt and challenges of their everyday. The ancient people were stimulated mentally and emotionally with all the dangers in the chase. How could they not be? They actually had the opposite problems to us. Never getting enough time to give themselves the mental and physical rest they needed to stay healthy, happy and strong.

Which leads us nicely to the "WHY" do we need exercise?

We have created our own problem here, simply by getting away from basic living, which involved daily physical output in return for food, living one with nature. Avoiding all the harmful toxins and additives found in our world and food. We don't hunt for our food and live off nature anymore.

We choose to eat processed foods with little nutrients, fill our bodies full of harmful Trans fat, which are WORSE than saturated fat, and to top things off we literally sit on our butts!

NEWSFLASH! Your body was designed to require and process specific amounts of lean protein, complex carbohydrates, good fats, various vitamins and minerals, AND regular cardiovascular exercise.

By not giving this to your body you're screwing it up. Sorry, there's no nice way to say it. If we want to live long, happy, healthy, productive, and fully mobile lives, we need to schedule daily cardiovascular activity to start.

You can choose to sit on your butt eating ding-dongs while watching life pass you by. Let the natural factors of aging slowly take your physical ability to move without pain away. Or you can stand up and fight it. By making a commitment to finding time to exercise and enjoy it, every day of your life. Time will pass you by regardless. And it's up to you to decide if you want to take matters into your own hands and make it better today than it was yesterday or not.

And I don't want to hear excuses, because experts agree that exercising in some shape or form benefits EVERY single being out there. Whether you have health issues or not, or your age number has crept way up on you. The pros of exercising outweighs the negatives. This is true even if you haven't exercised a day in your life.

The proof is in the pudding. I challenge you to do some "real" exercise and tell me, without pulling a Pinocchio, that you don't feel and "run" better as a whole!

We are going to look into the emotional, mental, and physical benefits of exercise in a broad scope. Starting with exercise basics, your body, and your thinking. We are going to have a look at how to prepare yourself for physical exercise. Followed by looking into some exercise lingo, workout ideas, and even some exercise equipment you may see fit to purchase for your quest of getting strong, fit and healthy.

FITNESS ALERT! Did you know that you are born with a set number of muscle and fat cells? So when you lose weight you don't lose fat cells, but rather shrink them when you send your fat packing. And when you are lifting weights, eating plenty of protein and gaining muscle, you don't create new muscle cells. All you are doing is making the ones you have stronger and/or bigger.

My thinking . . . I'm pretty sure you can see there are loads of reasons you are making the right choice to exercise. And I challenge you to give me a reason why you shouldn't be exercising. Exercise is fantastic for your mind and body. What I love most is the "feel-good" feeling you get when you are exercising and for a long while after. It's an overall sense of well-being, regardless of how your day has been going. Just knowing you are doing something great for you is reward enough.

Basic Benefits of Exercise

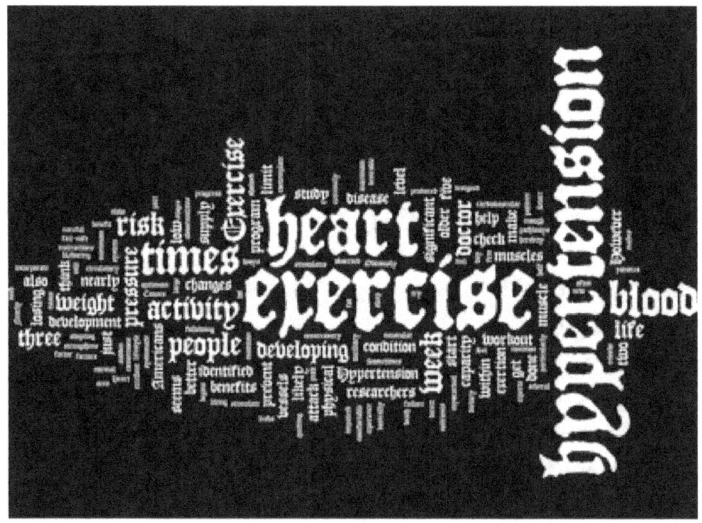

First of all I'm going to be the first to congratulate you on deciding to fit fitness into your life! Or perhaps just re-insert it? Change isn't easy and running a crazy busy schedule with so much to do and so little time doesn't help. I get it!

Here's a list of the basic benefits of exercise in a nutshell if you still need convincing.

MENTAL
- Better mood (natural endorphins)
- Increased self-esteem
- Better mood
- Higher feeling of energy
- Lower symptoms of anxiety and depression
- Better confidence
- Increased sense of pride
- Better able to deal with stress
- More of a level head in stressful situations

- Feel better about your look
- Feel better about the way others perceive you
- You'll feel better and trust more in your physical abilities

PHYSICAL/HEALTH
- Helps prevent annoying conditions and disease
- Lowers blood pressure
- Decreases the risk of heart disease and stroke and other serious ailments
- Lowers the risk of numerous cancers, diabetes, and osteoporosis
- Strengthens muscles, bones and supporting ligaments to decree falls and injuries
- Faster recovery time when injury occurs
- Tones and strengthens the body
- Weight loss
- Improvement in agility and mobility
- Less aches and pains
- Increased tolerance to pain
- Increased cardiovascular capacity
- Improved muscle endurance
- Lowers cholesterol levels
- Improves social benefits
- Improves circulatory function
- Improves skin, nails, and hair
- Aids in skin elasticity
- Decreases risk of back problems

Your health is important and the reasons above should be enough to convince you that any exercising is good exercising.

One thing I can guarantee you is that every little bit helps. And now that you know some of the benefits of sweating up a storm, you need to figure out what type of exercise works for you and find time to fit it in. If you like biking, then bike. If you prefer doing a group aerobics class, then that's what you should do. Experiment and figure out what works for you and get to it!

4-Another factor I don't want to overlook when considering a new exercise regime, is the inevitable fact of aging. The process in which our body naturally breaks down with time. One of the things in life we all have in common. You can choose to just accept the fact your muscles are going to break down, energy levels will start depleting, bones will weaken, and your skin will start to lose its vibrancy.

Or you can choose to fight the aging process and live a more fulfilling life longer. Getting yourself into shape and exercising on a regular basis is something you can do to help your body look better, be stronger, scare off disease, and make you feel better about yourself and life as a whole.

This process of getting fit is going to take patience, time, and perseverance. One step at at time. One foot in front of the other. Always looking to make better decisions and not being too hard on yourself when you take a step backwards. You're only human right?

All of this to better your health; mind, body, and soul. Giving you the opportunity to live a longer, healthier, and more vibrantly fulfilling life than you would otherwise. Opening the doors of opportunity that might otherwise have remained shut. That alone should be plenty to make you smile.

Be Prepared

* Stop and figure out what your fitness level is . . .

Before you decide to take on a new fitness routine, whether it's hiking, biking, aerobics, yoga, Pilates, boot camp training, or a gym circuit, it's important that you take a step back and measure your fitness level and knowledge. If you don't do this you could end up getting frustrated because you've picked exercises you can't do. Or maybe the level you entered was too high and you ended up getting seriously injured. Neither of which are going to help your head or your body reach your fitness goals.

A few factors to consider before you set foot into your new fitness endeavors are:

* Age - Sure, exercising was a whole lot easier in your teens. There weren't any aches and pains to worry about, and your attitude was that you weren't afraid to try anything. Invincible comes to mind here, at least for me. Well times have changed and it's important that you consider your wants and expectations, along with logic. I'm not going to tell you there is any particular exercise routine you can't do. But I am going to caution you to be sensible about it.

For instance, if you are enjoying your golden years and battling osteoporosis, you may want to steer clear of rollerblading, particularly if you've never been on skates before. That just makes sense, right?

Football is another exercise option that may have seemed awesome when you were 20 without a care in the world. But do you really want to sacrifice your body to get into shape, now that you are 50 with two young children? Probably not. So the point here is to think before you figure out what exercise options you're going to pick.

* Medical Conditions - This is a very important point. And for safety be sure you run any new exercise endeavors by your medical provider PRIOR to starting. It does you no good to start something, hurt yourself, and find out a few weeks later from your doctor that you never should have attempted it in the first place! Be smart and check first, just to be sure.

* Preferences and Tolerances - You know what you like and don't like when it comes to exercising. If you can't stand the thought of exercising in a gym, then don't buy a gym membership. Instead, you could join a cycling group or maybe try an outdoor boot camp. If you like the idea of working out with other people. Make sure you test the waters with some sort of group exercise class. Maybe you want to try kickboxing, aqua-aerobics, or a yoga class. The key here is to admit what you enjoy and don't enjoy, and set yourself up for success.

* Commitment - Getting into better physical shape is going to require a commitment. This means you sell yourself short if you only do it for a few weeks and then quit. Making a habit of being physically fit is something that takes time and patience. Give yourself a chance to get used to your new routine. If you do, it will be surprising how much more you come to like it. The rule of thumb with experts is 6-8 weeks minimum before you will start to get comfortable. Stick it out because the rewards are priceless!

* Don't Quit - If you are just learning the ropes in the fitness world and find yourself frustrated or bored. Whatever you do,don't quit! The only way this isn't going to work is if you walk away. It's better just to try something new. Maybe the cycling wasn't working for you? That's okay. Why not try getting a personal trainer or testing out the pool? Keep trying until you find the exercise niches that you really enjoy. Ones that you can see yourself doing for the rest of your life. Because that's what fitness is all about. A change for the better that sticks for the long run. Simply because you deserve to be healthy and happy, and live a long and productive life.

* Set Reasonable Expectations - Sure it's great to jump right into your exercise regimen. But if you overdo it you could be setting yourself up to fail. Many fitness beginners make the mistake of trying to do too much too soon. They are excited and hit the gym every single day for a few hours, thinking they

can keep this pace up. When they don't, these people feel down on themselves and end up quitting.

The solution? Slow and steady wins the race here. You need to take your time easing into fitness. Start with 2-3 days a week and work your way up. Consider your schedule and the longer term. By making sure you set reasonable expectations. You are one step closer to reaching each one of your fitness goals.

There's something really important I want to mention here just to make sure you've got the correct information. There isn't a doctor or health and wellness specialist out there that is going to tell you exercise is "bad" for you, regardless of your medical conditions. Fact is, the benefits of exercising outweighs the risks or negative effects, if there are any. Which is great news for everyone. Now this doesn't mean there aren't going to be limitations for some people with serious medical conditions, because there will be. But I'm going to tell you that with a little bit of effort there is exercise out there for everyone that will only make their situation better. Walking around the block, or even lifting soup cans for weights is better than nothing!

Make sure when you do start your new exercise routine that you begin slowly. Sure, you may be really excited to get going and that's great. But trust me on this one. Slow and steady wins the race. Too fast out the starting gates could lead to serious injury. And being sidelined for a few months isn't going to do you one bit of good when you're focused on finishing the race.

Fitness Alert - Did you know the best way to keep your energy levels up, especially when working out, is to eat smaller meals regularly? By eating five or six mini-meals throughout the day instead of two or three larger meals you are going to provide your body with the constant energy it requires to run efficiently. If you skip meals or only have a couple meals a day, your blood sugar levels are going to ride a roller coaster. This leaves you with energy highs and lows throughout the day.

Choosing smaller healthy food choices every two to three hours during the day will give you everything you need to keep your energy levels sky high for good.

My thinking . . . It's very important not to just jump right into a new exercise regime without thinking through the factors mentioned above. The idea is to make the best choices for you. The ones that are going to make you happy and get the results you expect and want. Where there's a will there's a way, and I believe you can make it happen. Just take it one step at a time.

Exercise Lingo

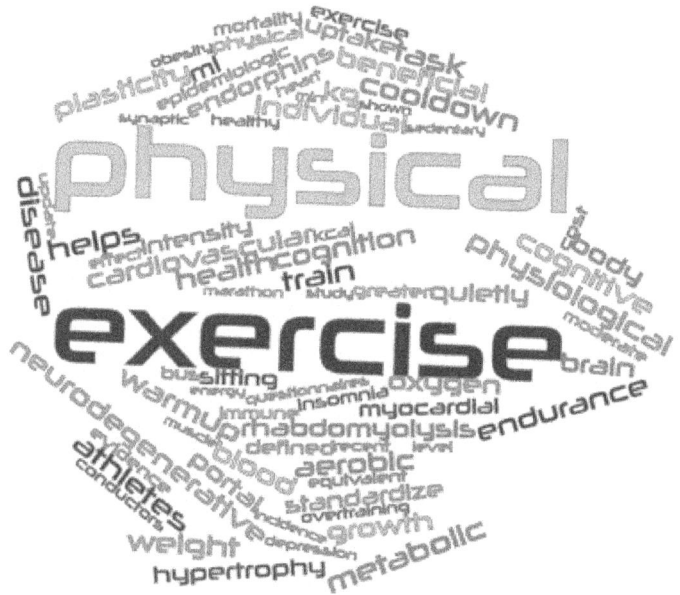

Unless you come from a fitness background, some of the lingo associated with it really is quite confusing. Well I'm going to help you nip this one in the bud by explaining some of the basic exercise terminology. By knowing what specific basic terms mean you are going to better apply them and get the job done right.

* Preferences and Tolerances - This just refers to what owning up to what you really want and accept this, gearing your new exercise program towards what you enjoy. Helping to set you up for success. If there is something you really can't stand doing. Then don't do it! Make adjustments around it. Perhaps you don't like lunges at all. Or maybe you have bad knees. So either do half squats or perhaps 1/4 lunges will work. And if you are

uncertain don't hesitate to ask a personal trainer. Better safe than sorry.

* Practicality - If you live an hour away from the nearest gym you have to ask yourself if you're really going to drive all that way for a workout after a long 12 hour shift? Maybe you could find a class closer to your work? Or perhaps you might want to invest in some exercise equipment to start? There's no use committing to exercising if it's going to be next to impossible to do given the parameters.

* Reps or Repetitions - Reps are a common term used to describe the number of times you repeat an exercise in one bout. Many people do 10 reps of a particular weight in each set, which I'll explain next.

* Sets - Sets are groups of reps. An example, there can be three sets of ten reps when executing biceps curls. This means you are going to do ten biceps curls in a row, and repeat this three times with a short rest after every ten reps. I understand this can be a little confusing at first, but it won't take you long to make sense of it when you are actually doing them.

* Rhythm - With exercising, this refers to the pace in which you are executing. So if you are doing squats, your rhythm may be in speed or count. Maybe doing three faster squats with a one count down and one count up. Then next time doing six squats with a three count down and two count up. What this does is keep your mind and muscles guessing, maximizing results.

* Weights - Weights are what you lift to work your muscles when you are working specific muscle groups. In the gym you will find weight machines, barbells, medicine balls and often kettle bells. These are just round bells with a handle, making them easier to grip onto. Weight training is used specifically

for muscle building. Helping you gain strength and burn calories more efficiently.

Fitness Alert - Did you know that muscle weighs more than fat does. As well, a muscular body is going to burn more calories than a fatty body of the similar dimensions. Which hammers home the point that muscle building is the right route to travel for a healthy, fit, lean, and energetic body.

* Muscle Building - This refers to focusing on building your muscles. Where you isolate a set muscle and work it specifically. Building muscle requires protein. Which is something you will need to eat 2-3 servings of each day, particularly when you are training, simply because your body can't produce protein, nor does it store it. And if you don't have protein available to use when you are trying to build muscle your body will break down the muscle you've already got for energy. Talk about defeating the purpose.

* Cardiovascular Activity - I think you know this one already. It's when you are exerting energy that gets your heart rate up, working hard to pump more oxygen and vital nutrients to your organs and bodily systems. It's also called aerobic exercise. Aerobic refers to "living in air." Which means providing enough oxygen when your body is exercising.

Examples of cardiovascular activity are:

- running
- biking
- hiking
- swimming
- aerobics class
- kickboxing class
- fast walking
- treadmill
- cross trainer

- skating
- circuits
- tennis
- soccer
- cross country skiing

* Interval Training - This refers to alternating bouts of high physical activity to levels of lower intensity activity. This can mean running for 3 minutes and walking for one. Or it can refer to alternating between weights and cardiovascular activity, intensity, and duration. With interval training you burn the maximum amount of energy in the shortest amount of time utilizing diversity.

* Maximum Heart Rate - Is the maximum heart rate your heart can reach according to your age and genetics. This is a safety measure taken when exercising to ensure you don't surpass your limitations. It's just a guideline and there are always exceptions to the rules. Knowing where your maximum heart rate falls will allow for you to exercise more effectively.

* Resting Heart Rate - Is the rate at which your heart beats at rest. Technically this means before you even move a muscle in the morning to get out of bed. Your resting heart rate will lower as you get in better shape. A great way to measure your fitness progress.

* Heart Rate - Is essentially the number of times your heart beats per minute (bpm) at any given time. For instance, your heart rate will be higher when your adrenaline is pumping, and lower when you are having a snooze.

Fitness Alert - Many people that are just starting to exercise are worried about getting their heart rate up too high. There are some pieces of cardio equipment at the gym that are equipped with devices to calculate your heart rate to ensure it's in the "safe zone." I would proceed with caution here because there have been numerous reports stating these readings are inaccurate. In fact, I have tested them on numerous occasions and found them to be 20 or 30 beats off.

If you are in doubt you can opt for the "talk test." When exercising you should be able to talk or hold a conversation with someone without having to actually stop to catch your breath. Unless you are in a specific training program. If you can't talk to someone while you are training, you probably want to slow it down a little just to be safe.

* Stretching - Stretching does not refer to reaching your arms over your head for 10 seconds. Rotating your arms around once or twice, and reaching down to the ground for another 10 seconds. Proper stretching will take at least 10 minutes and for good reason. You are trying to warm your muscles up to workout out. So you want them warm and "loose" so you will avoid injuring yourself before you even begin. On that note, you should stretch before and after every workout session.

Stretching is physical exercise where you choose a specific muscle group, tendon, or muscle to isolate and stretch or flex in order to increase the mobility of it. Just picture your muscle as an elastic band, and if you want it to stretch further you need to gently stretch it further bit by bit. Stretching should always be slow and controlled, never bouncy or jerky, and it shouldn't hurt. Each gentle stretch should be held for a 30 seconds to a minute and repeated.

* Forced Reps - The is a type of strength training often used in body building. Not something you will be trying anytime soon, but something you may want to tuck away for future use. Basically it's when your body has reached muscle failure when lifting. Which means you physically can't do any more reps. Of course you have a partner spotting you.

Instead of stopping you force yourself to do a few more, even though all your muscle fibers are telling you to stop. This is a shock to your system. You are forcing your body to stimulate more growth because you are now using muscle fibers that are rarely if ever used. This helps the biggest body builder to get bigger. And it's not something you do more than sporadically.

* Cool Down - This is where you slowly bring your heart rate down to your usual resting rate after exercising. So if you just finished an aerobics class. You might spend 10 minutes slowing things down to a nice walk, then do some gentle stretching, until you are totally cooled down.

* Warm Up - We touched on this a little already. Anytime you exercise, you should warm up. This is how you get your muscles and mind ready to work hard. So you might start with some jumping jacks and a light jog to get your blood flowing, letting your body know you are about to start exercising. In your warm up, you should include at least 10 minutes of gentle stretching. This will loosen your muscles and tendons and decrease the chances of injuring yourself.

* Rest - This isn't referring to taking a nap. A rest or break in exercise can refer to a stop between sets while lifting weights. Or a short break between exercises. It can also mean taking a break when training specific muscle groups. For example, you don't want to work your back muscles two days in a row. Normally no more than twice in a week is recommended for any one muscle group.

Rest can also refer to a break in training for your body to recharge and build muscle. This is especially important if you are training hard and lifting heavy weights. If you don't rest adequately you aren't going to get stronger.

* Supersets - These are another way to shock your system into giving you results when executing strength training exercises.

Typically this is a training method where you do two different exercises in a row with no rest in between, followed by a cardio activity. The idea is to alternate between muscle building and cardio exercises and keep your heart rate up continuously. This method is fast and effective. A great way to break through those inevitable plateaus where you just don't seem to be getting results.

* Upper Body - These are all the muscle groups above your waste. So your arms, shoulders, back and chest to start. Most people will strength train their upper body specifically one or two days a week, making sure they rest it in between.

* Lower Body - Are all the muscle groups below the waist. You legs and buttocks. The same sort of training regimen applies as your upper body.

* Core - Your core is a group of muscles that help to stabilize and move you different body segments. Think of it as the connecting factor between your upper and lower body. The groups of muscles in your core are your abdominals, hips and back. Having a strong core is important in preventing or minimizing back pain for example.

* Diversity - In exercising this refers in basics to changing things up. You see the more you diversify your workouts the more results you are going to get. By getting your head and body thinking, you will force maximum effectiveness in your training. In other words you won't be able to coast on autopilot through your routine without thinking. You will have to think about what you are doing with each exercise, which requires focus and concentration, maximizing your results and minimizing the time spent getting there.

A boot camp training session is a fantastic example because you combine a diverse range of high intensity interval training,

at your own pace, that's never the same twice. Always changing is great when it comes to fitness.

*Fitness Alert - If I had to choose one activity to challenge all
levels of fitness it would be group boot camp sessions. These
interval training sessions occur in a positive group atmos-
phere, driven by the energy of the room and the abilities of the
person next to you. These sessions are set up so that you challenge yourself to beat your personal best every time and
everyone is in the same boat, which is a motivator. It combines
a diverse range of cardio and muscle building exercises that
can easily be modified personally and still be effective. For example, if you have bad knees you don't have to do the squat
station, instead you can do ab work or pushups. And the in-
structors are always pushing and encouraging everyone to do
better. A fabulous way to get results fast, regardless of your
fitness level.*

*My thinking . . . It's very important to understand some of the
basic terms of fitness before you start to apply yourself. Yes, it
may be a little intimidating to start. But I promise you it won't
be long before you are used to most of the lingo used, and ap-
plying your new knowledge will be a piece of cake. If you don't
understand an exercise term, just ask!*

Workout Ideas

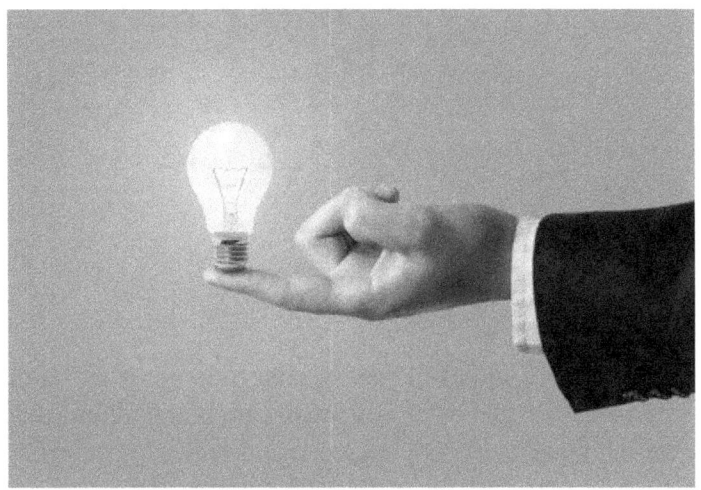

There are plenty of different workout options to help ease your way into fitness. One that you will enjoy and get results with. All you have to do is open your mind to all the different options, don't be afraid to try something new, and figure out what works best for you.

A few of the essentials in a complete body workout are:

* Stretching
* Aerobic activity
* Strength training

STRETCHING

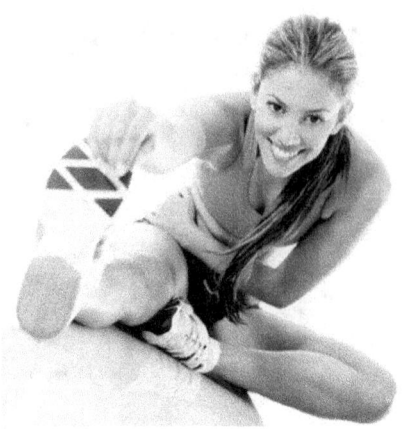

I know I probably sound like a recorder here but it's vital that you stretch before and after your workout, and even during if possible. Having your muscles loose and ready to perform is going to help you steer clear of serious injury.

Here are a few of the basic stretches:

Calf Stretch

Your calf muscle runs along the bottom half of the back of your leg. Very important for running, jumping, and even walking. To stretch your calf you can face the wall and place your hands against the wall in a pushup position while lunging your left knee forward with your right leg extended back behind you with both toes pointed forward. The idea is to gently straighten your back leg while leaning forward. Don't bounce or over stretch.

Hold each stretch for about 30 seconds and alternate legs 2-3 times.

Side Stretch

Here you want to stand sideways beside a wall. Cross your legs and place your left hand on the wall for support, while you extend your right arm sideways over your head towards the wall. You should feel the stretch up your side. Hold this stretch for about 30 seconds. Repeat with the other side and complete 2-3 times.

Quad Stretch

Stand beside a chair for balance. Stand upright with your hips square. With your right arm pull your right leg behind you up towards your buttocks. Make sure you don't lean forward here. Pull your foot towards your buttocks until you feel a nice stretch. Hold it for 30 seconds and repeat with other leg. Stretch each quad 2-3 times.

Hip Stretch

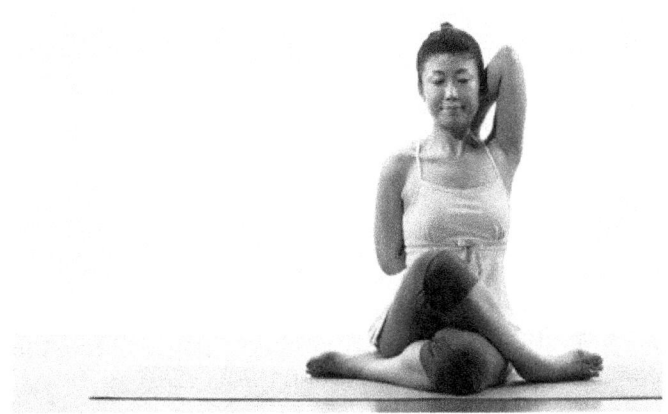

Sit down. Knees bent and cross your right leg over the left. Twist your body to the right and place your left elbow to your right knee, while twisting to the right. You should feel a gentle pull along your right side. Hold it for 30 seconds and alternate, repeat 2-3 times.

Hamstring Stretch

Lie down on your back with your feet close to a wall. With your left heel against the wall raise your right leg straight in the air and gently straighten until you feel a stretch along the back of your leg. Hold for 30 seconds, alternate, repeat 2-3 times.

Back/Shoulder Stretch

Stand with feet shoulder width apart. Clasp your hands together behind your back, bend forward at the waist and try and raise your clasped hands up towards the ceiling. You should feel a nice stretch in your back and shoulders. Hold for 30 seconds and repeat 2-3 times.

Head/Neck Stretch

Stand with feet shoulder width apart. With your eyes facing forward tilt your right ear down toward your right shoulder. You will feel the stretch along the left side of your neck. Alternate sides, hold each stretch for 30 seconds and repeat 2-3 times each side.

Knee/Chest Stretch for Lower Back

Lay on your back and bring your right knee up towards your chest while you left leg stays straight. Clasp your arms around your leg and I'll it in towards your chest. You will feel this gentle stretch in your lower back. Hold 30 seconds, alternate, and repeat 2-3 times.

Cat Stretch

This stretch will help to loosen you and get the blood flowing to your back, shoulders and core areas.

Get down on all fours. Arch your back up towards the ceiling like a cat while hunching your shoulders over and pushing your head toward the floor. Hold for 30 seconds. Then lift your head up, pull your shoulder back and push your midsection towards the floor and sticking your buttocks out. Hold 30 seconds and repeat both stretches 2-3 times.

Triceps Stretch

Put your right palm between your shoulder blades on your back, making sure your elbow is pointing towards the ceiling. With your left hand slowly pull your elbow towards your head using your left hand. Hold for 30 seconds and do the same with the other side. Repeat 2-3 times each side.

Bicep Stretch

Stand perpendicular to a wall at the end of it. With your right arm facing the wall, stand almost an arms length away and rest the fingertips of your right hand on the end of the wall. Twist your upper body gently to the left with your fingers still on the end on the wall, pushing your shoulder forward to feel a stretch in in your upper arm. Hold for 30 seconds, alternate arms, and repeat sequence 2-3 times.

Lunges

These will help stretch your legs. Stand with feet together. Lunge forward with your right knee, keeping your right leg straight behind you. Don't go past 90 degrees or you are over extending. Just lunge far enough forward to feel a gentle stretch. Hold for 30 seconds, repeat with other leg and complete 10 with each, and do 2-3 sets.

Stretching is something that will help you prevent injury and gain mobility and agility, along with improving your balance and coordination. There are lots of beginners stretching programs online to choose from. Or you can set one up with your personal trainer if that's the route you choose.

AEROBIC/CARDIOVASCULAR ACTIVITY

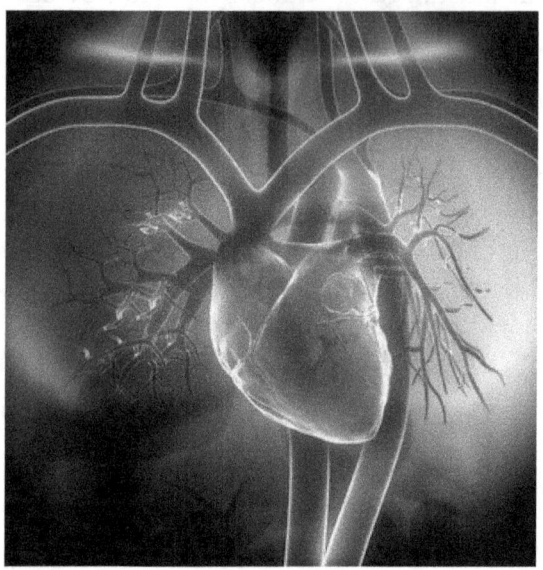

Improving your fitness level includes aerobic conditioning. Getting your heart rate pumping and blood flowing throughout your body. Transporting more oxygen, vitamins and minerals to your major organs and supporting systems, so that you can exercise longer and harder. Experts suggest you get at least 30 minutes a day of cardiovascular activity, with 45 minutes being ideal.

What's important here is that you think carefully before you decide on what aerobic activities you are going to participate in. Set yourself up for success and figure out what you enjoy. If you really loath the thought of committing to the gym and walking or running on the treadmill, then don't do it.

Instead, why don't you join a walking or biking group to start? If you work better with other people around as a support and motivator, then make certain that's exactly what you do. If you're pretty sure you aren't going to be able to motivate yourself to get out of bed every morning to go for run or hike by yourself, make sure you avoid this tactic.

It's also critical to note that you should rotate the kind of cardio you get each day. Three times a week you might do an aerobics session for beginners. The other days you might use the stepper or cross trainer at the gym, and go for a brisk walk the other days. Diversity is very important because it will keep you from getting bored and help you to get maximum results by keeping your mind thinking and body working different groups of muscles. Routine in fitness for beginners will take the wind out of your sails.

If you tend to veer off course you may want to consider hiring a personal training to set you up on a program that suits you. They will also make certain you get your butt to your training session. Definitely something to think about and worth every penny in my opinion.

Getting into great cardiovascular shape is going to help you to have more energy, see yourself and life more optimistically, increase your metabolism, flush toxins from your system, improve the efficiency of all your internal systems, and so much more. Bottom line is your body was made to exercises regularly whether you like it or not. Cardiovascular activity on a routine basis is a large part of it.

One other point. Walking around the block without effort at a snails pace DOES NOT COUNT as cardio activity. Nor does biking slower than a turtle. Cardio exercise to be effective requires effort. This means you should be working up a sweat. Not meaning you have to go so hard you are out of breath. But you do need to challenge yourself in order for it to count!

Here are a few great options for aerobic exercise:

* Biking
* Brisk Walking/Jogging/Running
* Swimming
* Hiking
* Gardening (fast pace)
* Aerobics Classes
* Boot Camps
* Treadmill
* Stair Climber
* Cross Trainer
* Elliptical Trainer
* Water Sports
* Soccer
* Basketball/Volleyball/Tennis/Hockey/Ringette
* Gymnastics/Cheerleading
* Yoga (specific types)
* Skipping
* Martial Arts
* Cross County Skiing
* Tobogganing
* Cross Fit

I think this gives you a pretty good idea what sorts of activities will get your heart rate up enough to qualify as a cardiovascular workout. Keep in mind that if you put an effort into things like housework and yard work, work up a sweat by keeping the pace up and your juices flowing, they will count as a workout. But it's up to you to either do it or don't. If you cheat you are only cheating yourself and your efforts in getting fit for beginners.

P.S. Sex counts as long are you're working hard!

STRENGTH TRAINING

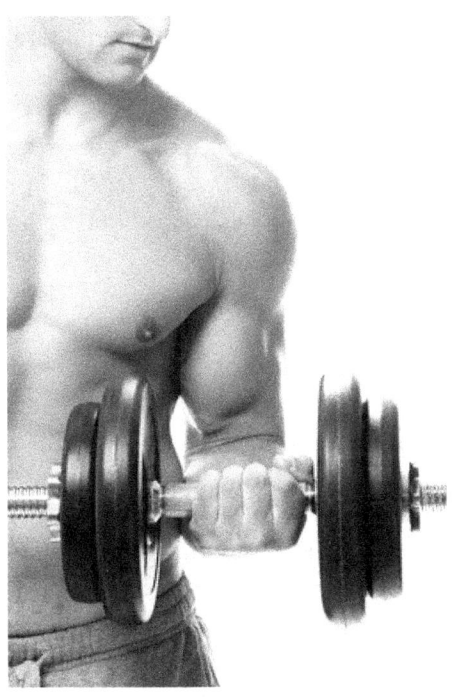

Your workout needs to have strength training of some sort. Whether you are working with free weights, weight machines, or resistance training, having strong muscles is important in your overall good health.

Strength training will help you feel good and look even better. It's a physical exercise that zones in on using resistance to force your muscles to contract, build strength, and improve the function of your body as a whole. As with any aspect of fitness for beginners, you need to figure out what works best for you. There are numerous options to help you build your muscles strong. If you have a job which requires a lot of physical effort, this can count towards your strength training. For example, farmers get plenty of muscle building every day working on the farm. From lifting hay bales and bags of feed, to moving heavy parts to fix machinery and lifting baby animals into their pens. If you work in a factory you may be required to sort and lift heavy objects all day, which should be considered strength training.

Lifting weights is the route most people choose when building muscles. You can choose to use weights or the machines to start. But a combination is best. Remembering that changing things up is only going to make you stronger, leaner, and get results faster.

We are going to focus on weight training and break it down into upper body, lower body and core. To start you can probably do a little of each. Simply because you won't be lifting heavy weights or doing very many sets with each exercise. Weight training is something you need to ease yourself into to avoid injury or just learning the wrong form/technique. Which of course will make your training ineffective.

After you get used to the weight training you might want to transition into doing upper body one day, lower body another, and core for the third day. With at least a days rest in between.

Upper Body

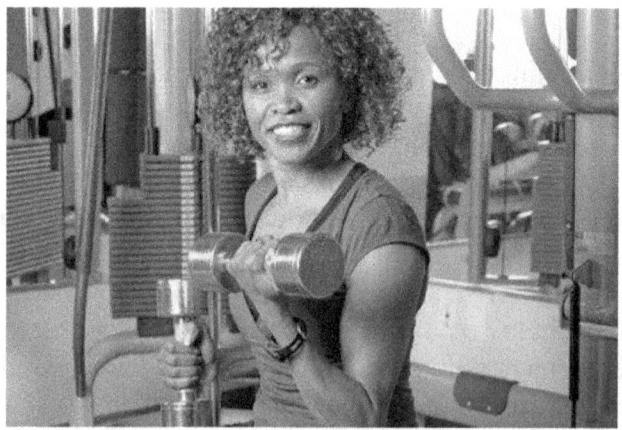

Bench Press

Here you are going to lay down on the bench with a dumbbell in each hand, making sure they are light to start. With your head looking straight at the ceiling and your knees bent comfortably and set on the bench, you are going to push the dumbbells up slowly and controlled towards the ceiling while breathing out. Do this for a three count. Pause and lower back down while breathing in, with a two count. Repeat this ten times, rest a minute and do two more sets.

Biceps

Stand feet shoulder width apart with a dumbbell in each hand. Your palms should be facing away from you. In a controlled fashion curl your left arm up towards your chest while keeping your elbow tight into your body and perpendicular to the ground, so it's just the top half of your arm moving upwards. Up for a three count and down for a two count. To ten reps with each arm, rest and repeat two more sets each arm.

Triceps

This muscle is along the back top half of your arm. Stand bent over 90 degrees at the waist with a weight in your right hand. Supporting yourself with your left hand on the bench or a chair. Bend your right elbow up and keep it parallel with the floor. Extend the weight backwards towards the height of your elbow, to a straightened position. Be sure to extend the weight upwards to make your arm straight. Don't drop your arm down. All while keeping your back flat and head forward. Repeat 10 reps, pause and do two more sets of ten. Alternate arms.

Shoulder Press

Stand with your feet shoulder width apart, knees slightly bent and weights resting on your shoulders. Push the weights upwards towards the ceiling up over your head, until arms are extended. Then slowly lower back down to starting position. Repeat this 10 times, pause and do two more sets.

This can also be done effectively with a shoulder press machine.

Pulldown

Here you sit on the machine and grasp the bar. Pull the bar down in a slow and controlled motion towards your shoulders. Pause at the bottom and slowly raise the bar back up to the starting position. Repeat this 10 times, pause and do two more sets.

Shoulder Fly

Sit on the machine, grasp the handles and let the pads rest on the top of your arms. Slowly raise your arms up so your forearms are parallel to the ground. Then lower back down. Repeat 10 times, pause, then do 2 more sets.

Lower Body

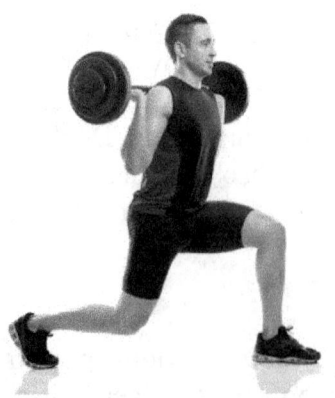

I would like to mention here that most cardio exercises work your lower body lots, so you may not have to focus as much here when it comes to weights. This doesn't mean you can ignore it, but if you only get two or three different exercises in when strength training, that should be plenty to start. Lower body training should happen 1-2 times a week.

Squats

I can't stress how fabulous squats are for working your lower body. Toning and strengthening your core, legs and buttocks. And when you execute this technique is really important. You need to ensure you stand with your feet shoulder width apart with your eyes forward. Start with a light weight bar across your shoulders, especially until you get used to the motion.

Keeping your back straight and butt sticking out, slowly lower yourself down to a 90 degree angle and back up again. This counts as one rep. Repeat this ten times, pause, and do two more sets. You should feel your thighs burning when finished.

Extensions

Sit on the machine and hook your legs underneath the pads. Slowly extend your legs up to a straightened position, and then back down to the starting position. Repeat this ten times, pause, and then do two more sets.

Hamstrings

Sit on the machine and place your legs on top of the pads. Slowly use your muscles to lower your legs down towards your buttocks. Then back up to the starting position in a slow and controlled fashion. Complete 10 reps, take a break and then do two more sets.

Core

There are literally hundreds of different exercises you can do for your core. We are going to have a look at a few to get you started. This core muscle group is actually known as your rectus abdominus, close to the surface of the skin.

Simple Crunch

The crunch will target the middle areas of your abdominals, around your navel. Simply lie on your back with bent and hands clasped behind your head. Slowly pull your chest towards your knees in a crunched position using your abdominals, slightly lifting your shoulders off the ground. You don't need a big motion to feel this one. Then lower yourself back down to the starting position.

Complete this 10 times, rest, then do another two sets.

Pelvic Tilt

These are great because you can do the anywhere. Lay on your back with feet flat on the floor, knees bent, and back arched. Place our arms outstretched to your sides, in line with shoulders. Breathe out and push your back flat against the floor. Be sure not to raise your hips up off the floor. Repeat 10 times in a slow and controlled motion, pause, and do two more sets.

Obliques

These core muscles help to bend your torso and rotate it. Lie on your back with your feet flat and knees slightly bent. Lift your legs off the ground, twist to the right and lower them but don't touch the ground. Ensure your arms are extended out to your sides and flat on the ground, along with your shoulders. Bring the legs back up to the start point and rotate to the other side. Repeat this sequence 5 times on each side, rest, and repeat one more time.

Lower Abdominals

Lie on your back with knees slightly bent, arms to your sides. Put your feet straight up in the air to start, lowering them slowly down towards the group until the touch slightly. Bring your legs back to their starting position and repeat 10 times. Make sure your motion is slow and controlled and bring them down to the count of three to start. Do two more sets.

Plank

This is excellent for all your core muscles. Lay face down on the ground. Lift yourself up off the ground, supporting yourself with your forearms. So up on your elbows if you will. Ensure your body stays straight and your core muscles and keeping your back flat and in line with the rest of your body right down to your toes. This is called the plank position. Hold this position firm for 10 seconds to start. Repeat this 3 times with a 30 second rest in between. As you get stronger lengthen the plank time by 10 second intervals. This should be challenging for you and if it isn't, you need to increase the duration.

Fitness Alert - You've got to start somewhere right? If you can only do a walk around the block a couple times then that's where you start from. As long as you are slowing improving, putting in the effort to build your cardiovascular capacity, then you are moving forward. Before you know it you'll be walking at a brisk pace for 30 minutes. It's all about progress and setting yourself up for success with REASONABLE expectations. The number one reason beginners fail in fitness is because they expect the impossible. Slow and steady wins the race here. Always pushing yourself gently to do more, and you will reach your goals - believe it!

My Thinking . . . Stretching is probably the most important as-pect of getting fit. If you don't stretch regularly you are going to get injured and sidelined, which doesn't help your fitness.

I'm a little bit different here because cardio is my favorite part of working out. It's where I get to get my heart rate working overtime, release my stress, and re-energize myself by tapping into my infinite endorphin stores. I can't tell you what the best cardio activity is for you. I don't know if you have any health conditions, if you're claustrophobic, or if out with nature is the only route to go for you. So it's up to you to try out different activities, even ones you "think" you won't ever enjoy, and fig-ure out what works for you. Aerobic conditioning can be fun and effective if you want it to be.

Of course strength training to build muscle is also very im-portant if you want to get strong, kiss fat goodbye, and keep it off by boosting your metabolism. Lifting weights for just 15 minutes 3 days a week is really all you need.

Equipment to Purchase

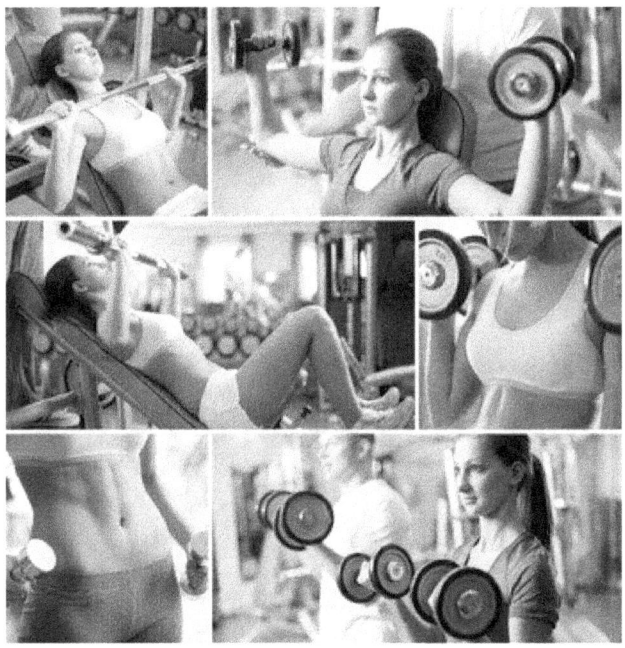

Fitness for beginners exercise routines are all uniquely different. It may make sense for you to buy a few pieces of gym equipment in order to get your workouts in. Especially if you are self-motivated and have a scary busy schedule. Which leads me to point that you don't need to spend an arm and a leg on equipment if this is the route you choose.

Garage sales are a fabulous place to get cardio equipment and weights dirt cheap. There's also the newspaper and often there are postings at local gyms. You probably won't be surprised to find lots of people that have purchased top quality equipment they never even ended up using. It's their loss and your gain.

To start, you need a piece of cardio equipment, and either some free weights or a strengthening device. Exercise balls and bands also work well. There are just so many options out there.

You just need to have a look around and figure out what suits you and your lifestyle best.

Here are a few pieces of equipment that are popular in a home. First we will look at cardio equipment, strength training, stretching and other.

CARDIO EQUIPMENT FOR HOME

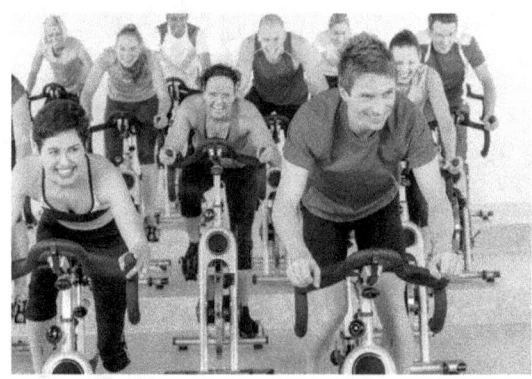

Treadmills

Good treadmills can be very expensive and really heavy. If you buy a cheaper one that's really light, I'm telling you now it will be a waste of money because they don't perform very well and just be a major headache. Trust me on this one. Cheaper isn't better with a treadmill. Before buying make sure you at least talk with a cardio expert from a sports equipment store. Combine that with the information you have and some internet investigation, and you will be able to get a great piece of cardio equipment to suit your budget and needs.

* Of course there's always your legs! Walking, jogging and running are all fantastic ways to get your heart rate up. And the best thing is you don't need any equipment, besides a good pair of running shoes.

Fitness Alert - I need to make an important point here. It's so very critical that you wear good quality shoes on your feet at all times. All sorts of health issues can arise from improper footwear. From simple blisters and calluses, to issues with your bones, muscles, and tendons, from wearing shoes that either don't fit or have the support your body requires. You are on your feet all the time, the least you can do is wear comfortable footwear that supports and fits your foot properly.

Ellipticals

This is a fantastic piece of cardio equipment that works both your upper and lower body simultaneously, with very little wear and tear on your joints. Nothing like running does for instance. Think of it as a cushioned motion that gives your heart a great workout. Most gyms have ellipticals, and understand it may take a few tries to get familiar with the motions. It will definitely test your coordination skills.

Having a piece of equipment like this in your home is likely going to cost you a little bit because the good quality ones are heavy, big and somewhat pricey. Just make sure you don't go cheap here. If it's too light you won't get the workout you need. Try a few out and make sure you speak with a fitness equipment expert before buying. I will say this is one of my favorite pieces. First prize for me goes to the spin bike thought, which I'll get to next.

Bikes

A very popular piece of equipment indeed. Most people can get their cardio on a stationary bike. Even people with bad knees and hips. Another plus is that stationary bikes aren't very pricy and if you find one at a garage sale even better. They are safer than regular cycling. So if you have mobility or balance issues for example, a stationary bike is an excellent option for cardio.

I prefer a spin bike myself. They are stationary bikes that are meant for hard riding, standing up on and moving around. These bikes are used specifically in spin classes which you may have seen running at the gym before. Other than boot camps, I believe this is the toughest cardio workout you can get. But the beauty of it is, you can go at your own pace. I love it fast and hard, so it works for me.

Stair Climbers/Stepper

These are pretty popular cardio in gyms. Recently prices have come down, which is great. But you still will need to opt for the higher end steppers and stair climbers if you don't want to waste money. The better models are heavier and well worth it. But you'll have to figure out your budget and what you are comfortable with.

Climbers work your lower body really well. Tightening your buttocks nicely for one, along with toning your thigh area. This is a great piece of cardio equipment to start out on. You can pick your pace and intensity level and work your way up.

Rowing

Rowers are another awesome way to get your cardio. They work both your upper and lower body effectively, and help with stretching, flexibility and mobility. The resistance and pace is set by you so you can start slow and work your way up. Rowing machines are fairly affordable which means you can get a good quality model without breaking the bank. This is the piece of equipment rowers in training often use off season.

Skipping

All you need here is a skipping rope and a desire to get sweaty. Skipping is an incredibly tough workout that takes time to master. If you can start doing 5 minutes, you are in great shape. This one is nice for the wallet because all you need is your runners, a skipping rope, and very little space. An excellent choice for taking when you are traveling and staying in hotel rooms.

Aerobics

Many people that are self-motivated will use aerobic videos to get a great cardio workout in. There are so many to choose from; kickboxing, hip-hop dance, and high-energy cardio. It's important that you get at least a couple different tapes if this is going to be your route. You always want to mix things up, otherwise boredom may set in. No matter your level, challenge yourself always.

Don't be afraid to combine two or three of the cardio activities. Maybe get one good piece of equipment, like a treadmill or stationary bike, and compliment it with a skipping rope and maybe a few aerobics tapes. The idea is to get your body sweating, have fun, and keep it diversified and exciting.

STRENGTH TRAINING EQUIPMENT

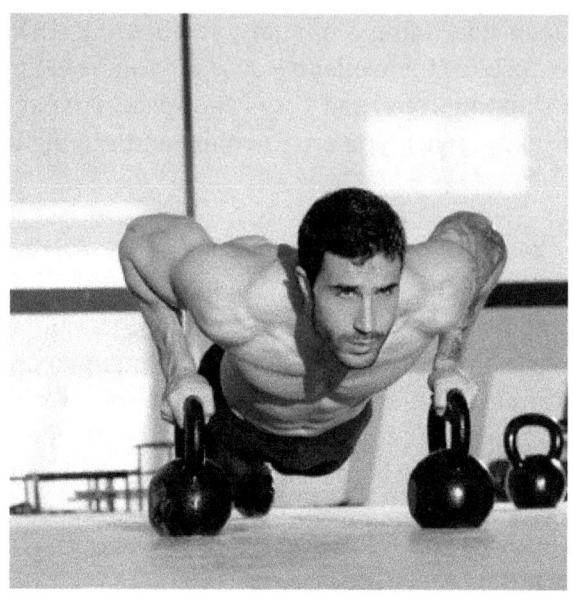

There are a whole lot of fantastic pieces of muscle building equipment out there, depending on your budget. You can spend very little, or a whole lot and get what you need to build your muscles and body strong.

Dumbbells

I would have to say these are something everyone has to have at home. Even if you are training elsewhere. With a few dumbbells you can work every muscle on your body. Starting off slow with the basic muscle building exercises for your upper and lower body. Then working your way up in variety, tempo, pace and rhythm. Each of these factors will positively impact your muscles, body, and overall workout.

The great thing here is they are cheap and take up next to no room. So you can even take them with you when you travel. Just 15 minutes three days a week is all you need to start building.

Home Gyms

Universal home gyms are another great choice that give your muscles a full body workout in the comfort of your home. Some use resistance and others have weights. Both are effective and you just have to test them out and figure out what works best for you. The price range goes from affordable to quite expensive, depending on your wants, needs, and budget. On a side note here. If you enjoy working out at the gym but can't because of your schedule or some other circumstance, a home gym may be perfect for you. They do take up a little bit of space, depending on the size you want, but definitely well worth it. To me it's diversity at your fingertips.

Resistance Bands

This is another great piece of equipment that's cheap and takes up almost no space. These bands usually come with sample exercises and can be used safely for building muscle while stretching. So they are fantastic for improving flexibility and mobility, so I'll mention them again when we get to that section.

With the bands you can shorten them more more resistance if you like, challenging your muscles more. And the great thing with these bands is you can set them at your level. Start off with little resistance and make sure your form is correct. Then you can kick it up a notch or two and start challenging yourself more.

Medicine Ball

These are great for building muscle and cardio at the same time. Depending on the weight of the ball you can do exercises to build muscle, or just make your Cardio activity harder. They don't cost a lot and it doesn't hurt to have them around to help change things up. Or just when you feel like working a little bit harder.

For example, if you are executing squats and getting pretty comfortable with them. Adding a medicine ball to the mix is going to give your mind one more thing to concentrate on and it'll get your heart rate up that much faster. In other words you're going to instantaneously make your squats more challenging!

Fitness Alert - Technique is everything when you are getting your body fit. If you perform an exercise incorrectly you are in danger of injuring yourself, and it won't be very effective. So you will be putting in the effort but not getting the results you want. This can be very frustrating and is often a factor that sways people to just give up. Start right and make sure you are doing the exercises correctly, and if you aren't sure just ask someone who's qualified, simply because it's very important.

Remember that you don't have to lift a lot of weight to build beautiful lean muscle. Which helps you look leaner and lose weight faster, because muscle burns more calories than fat does and actually boosts your metabolism. So even when you are taking a nap you are burning more calories than if you weren't lifting weights. Just 15 minutes about 3 times a week is all you need to start. Don't think about it, just do it!

STRETCHING AND OTHER

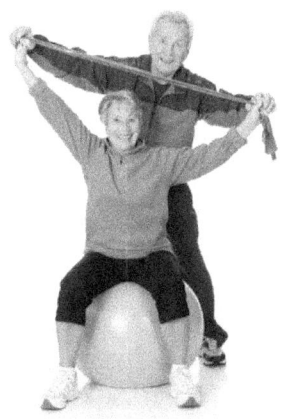

Here is where we are going to talk about stretching equipment and any other pieces you might like when you're about to engage in fitness for beginners. Remember, there are lots and lots of different stretching devices out there and you need to experiment a little and figure out what works for you. To start you just need your body, the knowledge, and the desire to get stretching. But if you'd like some equipment to motivate you or assist you, there's always:

Resistance Bands

Yes, we mentioned there above already, but resistance bands are excellent for stretching too. They will assist you in completing some stretches you might not be flexible enough to do right now. For example, there's a stretch behind the back where you try and reach your hands together. Most can't touch their hands. But using resistance bands will give you the stretch you want and help you to one day grab your hands. They also help you with form and give you a touch of resistance when stretching, which is going to build you stronger.

Mat

This isn't a must, but having a nice mat to stretch and weight train on, is always nice. It's good for your head too because it signals that it's time to get down to business, to focus on your training. Of course you can always use your floor, that works too!

Cruncher

There are all sorts of ab machines out there that range in price. A flag of caution here is to try them out before buying. More often than not you'll find that a diverse range of core exercises without equipment will do the trick to start. And when you get advanced you can always incorporate dumbbells into your ab routine, I love doing that. Don't be afraid to experiment a little, but always start off slow.

Exercise Ball

An exercise ball is great for using with weights, for core and stretching. It helps to add diversity in what you are already doing, and challenge you to push it to the next level. It's great for helping with form and supports your neck and back really well for core and strength training exercises. An exercise ball has just has so many different uses that I think everyone should have one.

Actual Stretching Machines

There are actually stretching machines out there that help you with your stretching, but they are fairly pricey. I myself wouldn't opt for one. If you are doing your stretching properly you really shouldn't need any equipment, at least initially. Maybe later on you will find a piece of stretching equipment that is helpful for you, and that's great. But I wouldn't go investing anything right now.

Weight Belt

Should you or shouldn't you? That's the question. A weight belt can actually get you into a whole lot or trouble injury-wise, because it makes you believe you have a stronger back and this makes you lazy in form. If you are lazy in your form you are going to injure yourself. So unless you are recovering from a back injury and understand the belt is just giving you a little more stability, I would steer clear of it. I'm sure you see some macho men strutting their stuff in the gym with their gynormous weight belt on. Chances are pretty good they're not even wearing the right size. Just be smart here please.

Ankle/Wrist Weights

You may or may not need these right away. But ankle or wrist weights are a great way to challenge yourself a little more. If you are wearing them when power walking for instance, this will take your cardio workout up a few notches. They are great for strength training too, just to give you a little extra. Always a good idea to have handy for when you need them. And they really don't cost very much or take up too much space.

As I've mentioned before, there are all sorts of tools you can use to help you get your body fit. It's up to you to decide how much you are looking to invest, and what your preferences and tolerances are. It kills me to see people unload lots of money on equipment that either lets them down, or they never really intended to use anyway. Just be smart here in your choices and buy only what you need. Test everything before you use it and when you do buy it make a plan to use it. You aren't going to lose fat, build muscle and increase your flexibility if your exercise equipment is dusty now are you?

Final Thinking . . . I'm not going to sugar coat anything here. Getting fit isn't easy, but that doesn't mean it can't be meaningful and fun. It may take some time for exercising to grow on you. So if you really don't "feel" like exercises for the first few weeks that's okay. But you're going to do it anyway. Treat it like a job and don't think about it so much. Just do it.

Given some time you will figure out what exercise routine works for you, your preferences and tolerances and limitations. And what you need to do is set your goals to challenge your limitations. Understanding that any sort of exercise is good for your mind, body and soul. It's going to help you build a stronger body and mind, feel fabulous about yourself, and decrease those pesky aches and pains you've accepted as "normal."

It's time for you to slip on your good quality runners and take the first step to bigger and better in everything.

Teaser to Book 2 - Pointers for Success in Health

What you eat is just as important as ensuring your body gets a good dose of exercise each day. Your body was designed to be physical, and in order for it to run efficiently and effectively it needs the proper fuel.

The right amounts of lean protein, complex carbohydrates, good fats, and essential vitamins and minerals to you stay healthy, energized and strong; mind, body and soul. Pointers for Success in Health is going to give you valuable tips in attaining great health and maintaining it, and so much more . . .

www.ingramcontent.com/pod-product-compliance
Lightning Source LLC
Chambersburg PA
CBHW070612290526
45790CB00002B/881